Faith That Overcomes

*How To Battle
Cancer and Win!*

*By
Patty Coons*

Bloomington, IN  Milton Keynes, UK

authorHOUSE®

AuthorHouse™
1663 Liberty Drive, Suite 200
Bloomington, IN 47403
www.authorhouse.com
Phone: 1-800-839-8640

AuthorHouse™ UK Ltd.
500 Avebury Boulevard
Central Milton Keynes, MK9 2BE
www.authorhouse.co.uk
Phone: 08001974150

First published by AuthorHouse 5/8/2007

ISBN: 978-1-4259-9533-1 (sc)

Printed in the United States of America
Bloomington, Indiana

This book is printed on acid-free paper.

Dedication

This book is dedicated to DeWayne, my husband, sweetheart, lover, encourager, and my very best friend who never let me fail. To my children: Sharon, Reneé, Kenneth, and Michael, who encouraged me by taking over duties at my home when I could not do it and did it without complaining.

I would like to express my sincere thanks to the staff and members of Faith City Church (formally Faith Fellowship Ministries) for their faithfulness in praying for me, ministering to me, and following the Lord's leading in keeping me optimistic. Thank you, too, Carol Baker, for your testimony that showed how God gave you victory over cancer.

I would also like to express my heartfelt gratitude to Ron & Cheryl Swift who stood with me during my trial by being there every time we called for help. No matter what time it was, they either prayed with us over the phone or came to the house personally. To Cheryl, also, who aided me by editing this book.

Finally, this is also dedicated to Dr. Karl Barancik, Pastor at Faith City, who took the Word of God and taught us how to live and use our faith to overcome the devil's schemes. Thank you, Pastor, with all our heart.

FOREWORD

By Dr. Karl Barancik

Christianity is unique to all other religions in the fact that it is based on God coming to man and changing him into a New Creation. 1st Cor. 5:17 says, If any man be in Christ, he is a New Creation". All other religions are based on man trying to get to God and please Him in some terms of personal acts. I have seen many people struggle with the Bible concept of a God that loves and cares about them and their woes. It can sadden a heart to hear God's accusers blame Him for every damnable problem, disease, and calamity that hits planet earth. But thank God that His plan for mankind was and still is a plan for good, with a hope, with a good future.

As a pastor for over 25 years I have taught that God's Word can be believed, confessed, and acted upon with great results. I have also watched God do special acts of grace and mercy on behalf of those who needed miracles. Over all these years of experiencing God's power and unchangeable Word, this I know, " God is a good God!"

That is what this book is about. A good God who proves that His Word can be trusted to change lives, heal bodies, and make the difference between life and death. What Patty experienced was nothing more that the divine Word of God spoken to create the final result that she expected. She found that God's Word never returns void or empty, but goes out to where it is sent, and makes the change that is asked for.

Patty writes about how God healed her of cancer, and what He can do for you. But please understand that Patty's victory came because she stood on the Word even when the circumstances said no way. She renewed her mind; dealt with negative thinking, keep her spiritual eyes on the prize, and won.

I want you to read this book with an open heart; open to God's miracle power that can change your life, just like it did Patty's. Let the following pages motivate you to grow your faith, because faith is our victory. 1 John 5:4 say it this way; "For whatever is born of God is victorious over the world; and this is the victory that conquers the world, even our faith." Enjoy.

PREFACE

"Fear not; [there is nothing to fear] for I am with you; do not look around you in terror and be dismayed, for I am your God. I will strengthen and harden you [to difficulties]; yes, I will help you; yes, I will hold you up and retain you with My victorious right hand of rightness and justice."

Isaiah 41:10 (AMP)

I wrote this book with the objective of helping women who are battling against cancer. I know there are many books out on the market about different people who have fought cancer. However, I never saw one written on a person's own experience. What actually happens to a person who goes through chemotherapy? What goes on in the body during this time? What goes on in the mind? First, listen to what the doctor says that is treating you. Be sure to get all the information up front from the doctor. If your doctor wants you to read papers on your therapy instead of explaining the treatments personally, find someone else. Be prepared and be sure to have a good Bible-believing church and people who will support you. This book starts out a little depressing, but I guarantee that it does not stay that way. Just be patient and keep reading.

My own personal story began in the early 1970's when I was just a teenager, and I was also engaged to my husband. My mother and my sister have been through removal of breast cysts. Unfortunately, I ended up having to have the same thing done.

My fiancée and I were new born-again Christians. We did not know much about the Word of God. We had older Christians who were disciplining us on our new walk with the Lord. It was fun and exciting. Both of us were on fire for God and wanted to learn more. After our marriage, we attended a spirit-filled, spirit-controlled United Methodist church. We were originally raised in the United Methodist Church. My parents were members of a church in one city. DeWayne's father was a United Methodist minister at another church.

During the recession in the 1970's, my husband got a job in Iron Mountain in the Upper Peninsula in Michigan where he relocated us. We attended an Assembly of God church there which we liked very much. At this time God began to develop our talent in writing plays. We performed a number of our own plays while living there.

After living in Iron Mountain the Upper Peninsula of Michigan for three years, we moved back down to the Flint area. We attended the Methodist church that my parents attended and worked in the church, joining the choir. A couple of years later I was asked to direct a choir at a Nazarene church. We attended that church for about 3 years.

During all this time, we kept questioning our religion and relationship with God. There had to be more than just living. Moreover, why did bad things happen to people? Where was God in tragedy?

There had to be answers. One night, we were watching television. We stumbled on a program that had a man named Kenneth Copeland speaking. We sat entrenched. He was answering all our questions. We learned that God had given Christians authority on earth to defeat the devil, to overcome sickness, poverty, depression. We did not have to put up with all the nonsense that the devil was dishing out. We so much wanted to find a church that taught the same thing. Our hunger for the Word of God grew, and we knew we had to get more instruction, but where?

We left our church service one night discouraged, because we were not being fed the Word of God. One day, DeWayne had passed a sign advertising a service being held at a church which was featuring Charles Capps, a minister who taught the Word of God like Kenneth Copeland. He was very excited! A church like Kenneth Copeland's, possibly. He had to check it out. I was pregnant with my son at the time and did not feel like getting out. DeWayne decided to attend a service to feel out this church. When he came home, he was so excited; it was all I could do to calm him down so he could tell me what he had found. He said that he had found our church. The Pastor of the church had preached the exact same message as our minister had done, but instead of condemnation, it was with love and the Word of God instead.

The Nazarene minister was leaving the church at the end of the month, so we decided it would be a good idea to leave at the same time. That was how we found Faith Fellowship Ministries. We have been members now for over 20 years. We also continued to write and produce plays. Suddenly, I was struck down with cancer with virtually no warning. What would we do now? How were we supposed to fight this?

Through the teaching at Faith Fellowship, we learned that the Word of God was our weapon. God had given us a way to fight. What was it Dr. Barancik said that was in the Bible? *"By whose stripes, ye were healed." 1 Peter 2:24.* (KJV) Thank you, Pastor, for obeying the Lord in preaching God's Word and praying for us. Without your assistance, we never would have learned how to stand on the Word of God.

Chapter 1

One morning as I was laying in bed, I found a lump in my breast. I thought, "Oh, no, not again! I just had a lumpectomy performed a year ago and now here is another one." The lump was on my right breast, between my breasts. It started out the size of a small marble and stayed that way for several months. After the development of the lump, I became tired, and had no energy at all. I thought maybe that I was weary because of a lack of exercise. Nonetheless, I ignored the feeling and kept on going. I did not want to admit that maybe the lump could possibly have something to do with it. After all, why would it?

All of a sudden, it got bigger. Within a week it swelled to the size of a quarter. I never had a cyst do that. Even though it was solid and hard, there was no pain. When I felt the new size, fear and worry entered my mind. I decided that I needed to get it looked at, even if it meant going through another lumpectomy, which I was not looking forward to having done. I had had two of them operated on over the years, and it was not enjoyable.

Just before I was married, when I was nineteen, which was about thirty years ago, I had my first breast cyst removed. At that time, there were no mammogram machines. The only way a doctor could tell for sure whether a growth was a cyst or tumor was to remove it.

Friday was the day the doctors performed this surgery. Women lined a whole floor of the hospital waiting for surgery — women who were scared, because there was no way of knowing whether their growths were tumors or cysts. All of us were wondering if we would come out of surgery still whole.

I hated hospitals. They made me nervous. When I was younger, I frequently returned to the hospital for different reasons. As a small child and not understanding what was happening, being in the hospital was not a pleasant experience. I did not like being put to sleep and then waking up feeling "like crap." So at nineteen, all I could remember of hospitals was that they were not a place where I wanted to be.

My roommate, who was a little younger than I, had two growths, one in each breast, which turned out to be benign. She did not communicate with me very much because she was so frightened. I went from room to room to visit with some of the women. Most of them were full of fear and worry. I was not too afraid because my mother had the same surgery done a couple of years earlier, and her cysts had been benign. I was sure it would be the same thing she had, and if all went well, I would be able to go home the next day.

Since the hospital was a training facility for student doctors, about twenty interns came and examined me. They would come in groups of three. They would smile and joke with each other as they examined me. The way they acted made me feel like this was their chance to handle women's breasts, and not for medical purposes. I was horrified. I felt like I had been molested.

They pumped me full of drugs to make me sleepy and to keep me calm. They told my mother that they had also given me a large dose of pain medication before I woke up. It was just a cyst, but the pain medication they gave me made me violently ill. I ended staying in the hospital longer because of it.

When I developed the second cyst about twelve years later, I was not looking forward to getting it removed. I did not want to go through the same thing as I had the first time. I was terrified. The memory of the first removal was still fresh in my mind. I did not have anything done with that cyst for about eight years because I was so afraid.

After my last son was born, we changed our personal doctor to a Christian family doctor. I was very comfortable with him, and he helped eased my fears. He sent me to his favorite surgeon — one he trusted implicitly. This surgeon and his nurse were also Christians. The cyst removal was performed in the surgeon's office. It made me feel better because it was more private, I did not have to be put to sleep, and my husband was able to be right next to me, holding my hand. He covered me completely except where the cyst was. This made me feel better because I wasn't exposed. Then he numbed me with a local anesthetic. The surgeon and his nurse joked and made small talk with us to help keep both of us calm, especially me. After he was finished, he gave me a chance to see the cyst. It was a large, marble-shaped mass of white flesh. I found it extremely fascinating. The doctor was confident that it was just a cyst. I felt like a heavy burden had been lifted off my shoulders. I felt ecstatic and overjoyed. I was free from the cyst and the worry that went with it. If it should happen again, I knew I would not be so afraid about having the cyst removed. The surgery had been an emotional and physical healing for me. The fears that I had had about the hospital disappeared.

Therefore, because of these two events, I was not too concerned with the third growth. We were attending a Word of Faith church at the time. I was determined that this time I was going to just believe God for the healing and not do anything else about it. I would go to prayer lines in the church, be prayed for by Pastor or one of the church leaders. One guest speaker even called out people who had some sort of growth to come forward. I did. However, in my times alone with God, He kept telling me to go see a doctor. I knew that meant seeing the surgeon who took out the other cyst. Finally, I agreed and went. (Never argue with God; we will lose every time.)

I had a mammogram which showed a mass on my right breast, but that did not surprise me because the last cyst showed up as a mass. As he had done before, the doctor did the lumpectomy in his office. This was on a Tuesday. DeWayne, my husband, was with me. However, this time it was different. The doctor had a hard time getting it removed. He had to keep digging deeper. This was starting to worry me. Some of the growth was under a muscle. He also had to keep giving me increasingly more local anesthetic to numb me. He said he had given me enough to numb a horse. Finally, when he was finished, he told me that it looked cancerous, but he felt that he had gotten it all. I felt a sudden streak of fear, but then it was gone and peace replaced it. The doctor said he would send it to the lab with a rush on it and let me know within a couple of days. The nurse was optimistic. She said she and the doctor would believe with us for the best, but if it turned out that it was cancer, I would need to go to the hospital and have more surgery. I was not a happy person. My feelings were confused and my mind was in a whirl.

DeWayne and I prayed together, believed God together, and read the Bible together. We found scriptures on healing and prayed for God's healing for me. I watched a video message by Jerry Savelle on standing and not giving up. He is a Bible teacher who is well known for his inspiring messages of victory and faith. His message was on fighting the devil with the sword of the Spirit, shield of faith, helmet of salvation, belt of truth, breastplate of righteousness, and feet shod with the Gospel of peace (Ephesians 6:14-17). He said we could quench all the flaming missiles of the devil. We can put this armor of God on so that we may be able to resist and stand our ground and then stand some more until we win. The message was very uplifting. I wanted to do this, but could it be this simple? For two days, I tried to believe that God would work everything out so I did not have to go to the hospital, but in the back of my mind, something was telling me otherwise. I knew this was not going to be as simple as the last lumpectomy. I dreaded the coming of Thursday. I hoped we would not hear anything from the surgeon's office.

Chapter 2

Thursday morning came, and I got a call from the surgeon's office saying they needed to see me. I was frightened, but did not cry. I called DeWayne at work and broke down crying while I was on the phone with him. He came home immediately after we got off the phone. DeWayne tried to calm my fears by telling me that I was going to get through this no matter what the outcome was. We both went to the doctor's office. He told me that the tumor was cancerous, but it was a type he had never heard of before. I could not even pronounce the name of it. It was a unique cancer, and he had to get a radiologist's interpretation of it. He said it was the kind that normally did not spread, and the survival rate was 99%. That was good news. However, the doctor wanted to do a bone scan and a CAT scan the next day regardless. Then I was to have surgery on Monday to go in and take out a little more tissue and to test my lymph nodes. Since the cancer had been against a lymph node, he wanted to make sure that it had not entered my system. My head was swimming with the report. Panic had set in again, and then it left, just as quickly. Even though the panic had left, my head was still dazed. It was like I was walking around in a hazy cloud.

That night at church, there was a prayer line right at the very end of the service. I went up to get prayer for good results on the tests the next day. The presence of God was so strong that I could not stay on my feet and ended up down on the floor. I was still on the floor when the service ended.

At our church we had certain couples that were placed over small groups of people. These couples were called Care-Net Ministers. They helped us, mentored us, prayed for us, and kept an eye on us. My friend and Care-Net lady, Cheryl, was praying for me. Suddenly I started coughing and could not stop. She and another woman were sitting next to me. I was coughing up "junk." I do not know how else to say it. They were handing me tissues as fast as I was filling them up. It was very bizarre. After about a half hour, it stopped. I did not understand what had been going on, but both of them were rejoicing and praising the Lord.

DeWayne took me to have the scans the next day. I was feeling very scared. I was to have the bone scan first and then the CAT scan. For the bone scan, they put me on a small table and strapped me down. This alarmed me, because I am severely claustrophobic. I was to be on this table for about 10 minutes under a machine that was inches from my face. I did everything I could think of to calm down, recite scripture to myself, even counting down the seconds turning them into minutes. The technicians would not let DeWayne stay with me for this scan. I was wishing they had let him, because it would have been easier to get through. Once the bone scan was finished, I nearly clawed my way off the table, but the nurse came quickly and took the straps off me. I was not sure how I was going to get through the next scan. I ended up having to take a mild sedative. DeWayne was able to be with me through the CAT scan. He held my hand, and I was comforted by his touch. I was able to keep a lot calmer. Once it was over, I broke down sobbing. All the emotion and stress that had been building up came spilling out all at once.

The surgery was scheduled for the next Monday in the late afternoon at the hospital. During the time of prep work and waiting, DeWayne read scriptures to me from the Bible. I was hoping the nurses would hurry and give me something to calm down, because I was so nervous. Once they did, it was easier to focus on what DeWayne was reading to me, which helped immensely. The nurses had me all ready to go when a tornado warning came across the public address system. A tornado had been spotted south of the hospital about ten miles away. Of all things to happen, a tornado warning! As if I was not all ready under enough pressure. All surgeries had been put on hold until the warning was over. My son, who worked at a McDonald's restaurant which was right next to the expressway, said he saw the tornado travel down the expressway and disappear out of sight. Finally, after half an hour, the warning was over, and I was taken into surgery.

I do not remember being put to sleep. It seemed like it happened so fast. The next thing I knew, I was waking up in recovery. I was feeling so miserable, doped up, and so sore, that all I wanted was my husband, but they would not let him come into the recovery room. I had to go back to the outpatient waiting area first. I did not want to move, but I knew if I did not, I could not have DeWayne next to me. That's why I made the choice to have them transport me, even though I felt I was nowhere near ready to be moved.

They put me in a wheelchair (even though I could not even hold my head up), took me to the outpatient area, and then put me in a recliner chair. All I really wanted to do then was lie down. They said when I was up to it I could go home. I just wanted to leave no matter how I felt or whether I was up to it or not. I wanted to go home and lie down and be with my husband.

After the surgery and while I was in recovery, the doctor told DeWayne that I was fine and that the surgery went well. They did not have to do a mastectomy. It appeared that he had been able to get all the cancer out in his office. They had removed some tissue, not a lot, and several lymph nodes from my breast where the tumor was. They also removed some lymph nodes under my right arm for testing. We found out later that no lymph nodes had been affected.

Chapter 3

A week after the surgery, we went back to the surgeon's office for a follow-up. He told us the results of all the tests on the tissues and lymph nodes they had removed. There was no evidence of cancer. It had not spread. The cancer was totally localized in the breast. The bone and CAT scans had also come out negative. I was fine. We were elated! It was over, so I thought. Then he said that I should see a cancer specialist to see if I needed chemotherapy because of the size of the lump. I suddenly felt very light-headed, like I was in a far off place.

The surgeon sent us to an oncologist. The doctor met us in his office. My mind was still reeling, so I had to depend on DeWayne to listen to the doctor and tell me anything I did not understand. What I could understand, though, was why the doctor did not seem together. He kept looking back at my chart and looking up notes on what he should do. He acted as if he was completely at a loss as to what procedure he should take. Then, in the middle of the session, he stopped and talked to a physician over the phone about another patient. We were rather embarrassed because we knew the person he was talking about. At the end of the consultation, he had me go into a diagnostic room where he examined me without letting me put on a gown. He tried to push my breast out of my bra. When he failed, because he was hurting me, he finally undid it. DeWayne was very offended, but before he could do anything, the doctor had me most of the way undressed on the top. I was so out of it that I did not react to the way the doctor was treating me. I just sat there dumbfounded, not knowing what to do. Afterward the doctor left the room with the door opened and me exposed. DeWayne quickly shut the door and helped me get dressed. He took my arm, and we met the doctor back in his office. He proposed to do six chemo treatments followed by radiation. He said that I would lose my hair. We asked for a week to think about it. I felt completely lost.

At home that night, we talked about the oncologist. We were very upset about the whole meeting. DeWayne said he had counted nine times when the doctor had to look up the same information on how big the tumor was as well as other details. He really seemed confused and unable to remember. He was not sure about what treatment to give me; he kept looking through a medical book and going back and forth on what he was going to do. He said the tumor was four centimeters in size. His book said <u>not</u> to use chemo for three centimeters and under, but to use chemo for five centimeters and over. He kept rereading the section as if he was uncertain on what to do at four centimeters. We were not comfortable with him. I was glad that DeWayne had been paying attention to what had happened, because I was so overwhelmed by everything that I was very despondent and could not even think straight.

At the oncologist's office, I had been given the name of a hair stylist who sold wigs. The hair stylist specialized in working with chemo patients. She was wonderful. Even though I was feeling depressed and still muddled up, she tried to help me relax by having a happy attitude and telling me funny stories. At the same time, she explained how to style my wig and wear different scarves and hats to help me cover my soon-coming lack of hair. She also kept telling me not to worry, that this was only temporary, and that my hair would grow back. In fact, she said, it would most likely grow back thicker, wavier, and softer. I did not see how that was possible. The thing I knew for sure was that I was very self-conscious about possibly not having any hair, and I wanted the wig as close to my natural color and style as possible. She matched my hair color exactly and ordered the wig. Once she got it, she styled it to the appearance and length of my hair. It was beautiful and made me feel a lot better.

Chapter 4

The next Tuesday my mother, who was 79 years old, passed away. My mother and I were very close. Both of us felt that we could talk to each other about anything, whether it was problems or just small talk. The last three years of her life, her health deteriorated rapidly. It was very difficult to see a person that I loved so much waste away. She had suffered two major strokes and then several small strokes over the course of five years. We decided to move together in homes across from each other so my family could help her out if needed. We had lived that way for about two years, but my two daughters (who were in their early twenties) finally had to move in with her to take care of her. They were perfectly willing to do this — in fact; they volunteered. However, her last six months, she had gotten so bad that my daughters could no longer assist her. Since I held power of attorney, I had to put her in an assisted living home, but she had had a massive heart attack while she was there, and the home could no longer give her the attention that she required. Because of her history, there was nothing the doctors could do for her, Therefore, I had to move her to a nursing home to get twenty-four hour supervision. She was only there for a month and a half.

When the phone rang about two in the morning, I knew instantly it was the nursing home. One of the nurses told me that she had passed on. Even though I knew she did not have much time left, it still hurt to have her gone. DeWayne held me until I stopped crying. I then called my sister who lives in Maryland and my brother who lives in Florida to let them know.

I never told my mother about what I was going through. She was too ill, and I did not want her worrying about me. Before she died, I had my hair cut short, because the doctor said the treatment would make me lose my hair. When I visited her, I just asked her if she liked my hair cut. She nodded. My hair, before it was cut, ended at about the middle of my back. It had taken me a long time to get it this length. I was not happy about cutting it short or possibly losing it all together. In fact, it made me angry. I did not want this to happen.

DeWayne and I went to see my mother right after she passed on at the nursing home. I wanted to see her before the funeral home took her away. She looked at peace. Through my tears, I asked the nurse what happened, and all she could say was that she had looked in on her an hour before. When she looked in on my mother the next hour, she was gone. Neither one of us had gone back to sleep that night. Once morning came and I knew everyone would be up, DeWayne and I spent the day making arrangements. The funeral was going to be the following Monday. This was just one more anxiety that I did not need.

A few days after the funeral, my sister wanted to go visit mom's grave before she went back to Maryland. She talked to me while we sat under a tree near my mom's grave. She asked me about my health and questioned me on whether I had lost weight. I had not lost any weight, but apparently I was still pale from the surgery. She said several cousins had asked her too. I tried real hard to be lighthearted and told her I was fine and that I still weighed the same as I did after my last baby was born. I could not tell her what was really going on. I felt she did not need to know, being so far away. There was not anything she could do anyway. Even though I wanted so much to confide in her and tell her my heartache, I did not want her worrying about me, either.

Chapter 5

We saw the oncologist a second time, and again he discussed another patient's medical history in front of us with his dictation recorder. He also did not seem to remember the earlier visit that he had with us. At this point, both of us were extremely frustrated and disillusioned. That evening, DeWayne and I discussed the doctor's behavior again and made the decision that I was not going to be treated by this oncologist. He was not dependable. We made an appointment that Thursday with the surgeon, who had referred us to this oncologist, to discuss what had happened at the oncologist's office. The surgeon was real disappointed in the doctor's behavior, but then told us that his wife had left him just a couple of days before our first visit and had taken all the furniture from their home with her. Nevertheless, he said that still was no excuse for his behavior. He should not have acted like that. The surgeon decided right then to send us to another oncologist. This one was a little closer to our home.

We talked to this doctor and told him about the first oncologist. He promised he would take real good care of me. He changed the treatment a little, wanting to use a different chemo mixture followed by radiation. He was not very thorough about explaining everything, but we liked him a little bit better than the other one. I was to have one chemo treatment every three weeks. A nurse gave me a bunch of papers and told us to read them. After everything that I had already been through, I was not in any kind of shape to read papers on cancer. DeWayne glanced through them.

The nurses scheduled an outpatient surgery to put a passport in my arm so the chemo would be fed directly into a main artery near the heart. That way the chemo would not damage the veins. The passport was a small device that would be placed under the skin of my left arm. I knew very little about it at this time. Another procedure to go through that frightened me. I was having so many anxiety attacks, that I depended on medication to keep me calm. Since I could not eat or drink anything, that meant I was not able to take my medication. The nurse, however, gave me morphine to calm me down, for which I was very grateful. Once in the same surgery room, the surgeon that put the port in was not very talkative or friendly. He seemed preoccupied and was not interested in conversation. I tried to get him to explain to me what it looked like and how it worked, but he kept to himself and just did the job. The atmosphere in the room was very gloomy.

I also had to have a heart test (a name too complicated to pronounce) to determine how much chemo I could handle. This was done at the same place where I had the CAT and bone scans. Once again, I had to lie on this small table while this big machine took pictures of my heart from two different angles. The nurse could not figure out why my heart was beating so fast. DeWayne was able to be with me this time. He told her that I was claustrophobic. She assured me that it would not take long, but I still did not like it.

During this whole time, DeWayne, of course, had to take time off work to be with me at all these appointments. He was not about to let me go through this by myself. When he told his boss what was going on with his wife, his boss told him to take as much time as he needed to be there for me. DeWayne is very valuable at work because of his skill in computers. He can fix and reprogram almost any computer. Where he works, his office services computers for many different companies. They did not want to lose him just because he had to take some time off work to be with me. He was too important to the company.

Chapter 6

The day finally came for my first chemotherapy. I was not looking forward to it. All this time, DeWayne and I had been praying and reading the Bible together before bedtime. We were praying for God's healing through the work of the medicine. We found different verses in the Bible that we claimed for me. (I have included some of those in a later chapter.) The doctor and nurses said I should not have any problems as long as I took the four different kinds of anti-nausea medicine to keep me from getting sick to my stomach. I took them before I left the house.

We tried to get the doctor to tell us what chemotherapy medicines I was going to have, but he would not tell us. All he told us was about some chemical called FEC, whatever that was, but he never told us the dosage. He just wanted to give it to me. He did not want to be bothered to explain the procedure, just that I would have six treatments. I know that DeWayne was a bit annoyed with the doctor. I was too whacked out to know up from down.

The treatment was on a Thursday and took three hours. I was there most of the afternoon. The room was lined with recliners with an IV pole by each chair along with a waste can for hazardous material in which the nurses threw away needles, IV bags, etc. It was not a very positive or pleasant atmosphere. I was given numbing cream to put on my arm where the passport was so it would not be painful to put in the IV. The chemo was given through an IV bag along with huge syringes the size of milk bottle caps and as long as a six inch ruler. The nurse gave me more anti-nausea medication that made me sleepy. I slept for a few minutes but not long. A lady next to me noticed I was awake and asked me if this was my first time. I said yes. She said I would probably lose my hair but that it was ok, because it would grow back. She said just have myself a good cry and try not to think about it. I think she was trying to reassure me by continuing to say that this was not the first time she has had to have chemo. She mentioned that she had her cancer come back about three times now and having chemotherapy was no big deal. Everything around me, the room, the nurses, the other patients, was just so negative. The oppression in that area was so heavy with the spirit of death, it was almost felt in the air.

After I got home, initially, I felt all right and even ate a light supper. However, about two hours later, I got very ill. I could not keep anything down. Hour after hour, I was throwing up. It was really making me nervous. DeWayne made me a bed on the bathroom floor because I was too weak and sick to go back to bed and then try to run back to the bathroom again. He lay there with me in case I needed help. DeWayne had called the doctor, who did not seem to care when he told him how ill I was. He just told me to keep taking additional doses of the nausea medication. It did not help at all to stop the nausea. After six hours of this, I finally ended up going to the hospital during the middle of the night to get something to stop the queasiness. The doctor gave me something through an IV to settle my stomach. It worked, but made me very sleepy. After several hours there, I was released and sent home. I was no longer vomiting, but my stomach was very upset. I had to keep taking the nausea medicine for the next two days to even keep water down. It was about four days before I was able to eat anything.

After the weekend, the doctor's office tried to give me something else to help keep me from getting sick to my stomach, but it did not work. It was the same type of medication but just in a different form. I was also to go in to get shots that were to raise my white blood count back up, because the chemo would lower it. It was standard treatment to get five shots. I may even need a shot to raise my hemoglobin depending on how low the chemo decreased it. However, after a week, my counts were still low. This was unusual, so I needed more shots. The doctor did not believe me when I told him that after a whole week had gone by, I was still ill. This entire episode was enormously exasperating! I was getting very infuriated with the doctor for not believing me. Finally, after about two and a half weeks, my appetite came back, and I was eating again. I felt enormously ecstatic. I had lost five pounds. Probably to anyone else, five pounds does not sound like much, but I only weighed a hundred and fifteen pounds and was tall and slim. I have to fight to gain weight and to keep it.

The next week I started running a fever. The doctor on call put me in the hospital for fear that I had developed some sort of infection. I knew that it was just a cold, but because my white count was so low, I could not fight it off myself. Being in the hospital had made my condition worse. I was fighting fear as well as sickness. Nearly all of the nurses were wonderful in caring for me, but I could not stop the anxiety attacks. Because of this, I could barely eat. Most of my food was left untouched.

The fever finally broke, but I was worn out. I had drenched my gown and bedding. The nurse came when I called and changed the sheets and me. The next day we received the report that all the tests they ran on me in the hospital came back negative, no infection. When they finally released me five days later, I had lost a lot of my hair on the back of my head and my weight had dropped fifteen pounds.

I went back to the oncologist for a check-up. It had taken ten shots instead of five to raise my white count up and two shots to bring my hemoglobin back up. I should not have had to have any more than five. Most patients did not need to have that many shots. The chemotherapy had been excessively strong for my system. I was so depressed with everything that had happened, the doctor put me on an antidepressant, Zoloft. He gave me time; it was up to me to decide on how long I felt I needed to get my strength back before the next treatment.

After a month and a half, I gained some weight and strength back. My hair, however, was coming out in clumps. But I was not going to let satan get me upset about my hair. Again, during this time, DeWayne and I kept praying and reading the Bible together with the same prayers and scriptures. DeWayne's support during this time was very important. He kept encouraging and supporting me. He told me he did not care if I had hair or not. That was not the reason why he loved me. Hair or not, he was happy to have me alive; nothing else mattered. His support helped keep me energized. The two of us were in agreement, *"Again I tell you, if two of you on earth agree (harmonize together, together make a symphony) about — anything and everything*

— whatever they shall ask, it will come to pass and be done for them by My Father in heaven." Matthew 18:19 (AMP) became a very strong bond for us. I ended up wearing a wig when I was outside and a turban in the house, because the wig was too hot to wear constantly. The turban covered my head completely. At night, I had a sleep turban to put on my head. Having these three items made enduring my hair loss a lot easier and I was less self-conscious. No one would see my baldhead and I was not going to let anyone see me without my hair including my children. DeWayne was the only one I permitted to see me that way.

Chapter 7

The time came when I knew I had to continue the treatments. I was not thrilled about going through another round. In addition, during this time, satan kept bringing to my mind people and friends who died of cancer. Every time I turned on the TV or read a magazine or newspaper, someone had died of cancer. Television can be a very powerful tool of the devil's and he likes to use it. Then of course, satan would remind me of my mother and what she looked like in her casket. It was so eerie and dismal. Everything around me was destructive and devastating. Even though the surgeon said I had a 99% chance of survival, the devil was telling me otherwise. My head was so befuddled; I had a hard time controlling my thoughts. However, I knew enough to never speak out those things that had entered my mind.

The antidepressants were helping me out of the depression that had set in and, with the prayers of others, the words of my Pastor and God's Word were starting to take effect in my mind. Gradually, I started to revive a bit. I was getting stronger in my mind. I had to make a decision where my life was going to go. DeWayne and I worked together in agreement for my healing, and I was not going to give up. These verses became my anchor:

"Grant you according to your heart's desire, and fulfill all your plans. We will (shout in) triumph at your salvation and victory..."   Psalms 20:4-5 (AMP)

"The king [David] shall joy in Your strength, O Lord; and in Your salvation how greatly shall he rejoice! You have given him his heart's desire, and have not withheld the request of his lips. Selah [pause, and think of that]! For You send blessings of good things to meet him; You set a crown of pure gold on his head. He asked life of You, and You gave it to him, long life forever and evermore. His glory is great because of Your aid; splendor and majesty You bestow upon him. For You make him to be blessed and a blessing forever; You make him exceedingly glad with the joy of Your presence. For the king trusts, relies on and is confident in the Lord, and through the mercy and steadfast love of the Most High he will never be moved."

Psalms 21:1-7 (AMP)

"Fear not; [there is nothing to fear] for I am with you; do not look around you in terror and be dismayed, for I am your God. I will strengthen and harden you [to difficulties]; yes, I will help you; yes, I will hold you up and retain you with My victorious right hand of rightness and justice."   Isaiah 41:10 (AMP)

"But He was wounded for our transgressions, He was bruised for our guilt and iniquities; the chastisement

needful to obtain peace and well-being for us was upon Him, and with the stripes that wounded Him we are healed and made whole."   Isaiah 53:5 (AMP)

"...yet My love and kindness shall not depart from you, nor shall My covenant of peace and completeness be removed, says the Lord, Who has compassion on you."

Isaiah 54:10 (AMP)

"You shall establish yourself on righteousness — right in conformity with God's will and order; you shall be far even from the thought of oppression or destruction, for you shall not fear; and from terror, for it shall not come near you."   Isaiah 54:14 (AMP)

"But no weapon that is formed against you shall prosper, and every tongue that shall rise against you in judgment you shall show to be in the wrong. This [peace, righteousness, security, triumph over opposition] is the heritage of the servants of the Lord...."

Isaiah 54:17 (AMP)

"So shall My word be that goes forth out of My mouth; it shall not return to Me void — without producing any effect, useless — but it shall accomplish that which I please and purpose, and it shall prosper in the thing for which I sent it."   Isaiah 55:11 (AMP)

I personalized these scriptures, put myself, my name in them, and said them every day. I had to. There was no choice in this matter if I wanted to win.

Chapter 8

Once I made the decision to win, not give up, and speak only God's word, God then started showing me people who had survived cancer. Every week someone else came to mind that was still living and no longer had cancer. God even used the television to bring positive images to my mind. One lady in the church took me aside and said that she had had breast cancer several years ago. Her cancer had been a lot worse than mine. Now she was fine, no more cancer and stayed cancer free for many years. She was a sustaining figure for me. I had people in the church besides my Care-Net couple that was supporting me. In addition, my video department team, of which I was director, was also supporting me. They kept the cameras and tapes rolling even though I could not be a part of them at the time. My other two directors helped me by working extra times until I could come back. I was experiencing contentedness and optimistic. The one thing I did not want to do was to go back to the oncologist's office.

After a month and a half, DeWayne and I decided it was time to see the oncologist. He said he would cut the treatment in half, not give me as much chemo, and eliminate one of the drugs. He said that another patient had similar problems, and when he had eliminated the third drug, she stopped being ill. Therefore, I had the second treatment. This time, it did not take three hours. The doctor did reduce the chemo.

That evening, however, I still got ill and, following the doctor's instructions, began to take additional doses of the various anti-nausea drugs he had given me. I was able to keep from vomiting, but instead began to have convulsions. I could not stop shaking. DeWayne said that at times my eyes would roll back into my head, my tongue was hanging out, and my back was arched. He called our Care-Net couple. They came over right away and prayed for me. The convulsions finally slowed and stopped. I was exhausted, in pain, and scared. During the prayer, God had talked to DeWayne and told him that it was one of the anti-nausea medicines that was the cause of the convulsions. Consequently, he went out on the Internet and checked on the drug. Sure enough, it said that when taken in combination with two of the others drugs I was on, it can cause shaking. I stopped taking the medicine and had no more trouble with convulsions. I had had nothing like that happen to me before, and it was dreadfully disturbing.

The next check-up we told the doctor what had happened. We told him that I had not been sick, but had convulsions instead and that we had traced the problem to the one anti-nausea drug. His reaction was, "Why were you taking that drug?" However, he was the one that had prescribed it in the first place. I was baffled! Why would he say that?

Because I was still so sick, weak and unable to eat for nearly a weak, the doctor said he would give me even less chemo in the next

treatment to try to get my nausea under control. Again, we tried to get
him to tell us the dosage of the medicines that he was giving me. He
assured us that the dosage would be "less", but would not give us exact
numbers or details. We left with more questions than answers. What
in the world was going on?

When I went in for the third treatment, I asked the nurse as she
was administering the medication how much the doctor had reduced
it from the last treatment. She seemed surprised by the question and
told me that I was getting the same amount I had received the last
time. The doctor came into the treatment room at that moment, so my
husband and I asked him about the dosage. He insisted he had reduced
the dosage. By now, DeWayne was getting tremendously impatient,
and continued to pressure him for exact numbers. The doctor checked
my chart and finally gave us the original dosages of my first treatment
and what I was receiving now. He had told us that he had reduced
my dosage "by half", but the numbers he gave us did not show that he
had.

I then informed him that I would have to move the next treatment.
My older son, who was born with a cleft lip and palette, was scheduled
to have surgery at a university hospital, which was about an hour away
the day after my next chemo. My son had had several surgeries before
this to correct the birth defect. This one was to straighten his crooked
nose. I did not think I would be able to have a chemo treatment one day
and be able to recover enough to handle the hospital trip the next day.
The doctor then berated me for having been so sick and told me I had
better stop doing that. There was nothing wrong with the treatment I
was receiving, and I was only getting sick because I wanted to be sick. If
I did not want to be sick, I should just stop being sick. I should be able

to have the treatment and still handle everything else the next day if I just wanted to do it. He would not permit me to reschedule the chemo treatment. This upset me greatly, and I was getting livid.

DeWayne then tried to ask him why the numbers did not match his statements about my dosage and why the nurse was telling us something different than he did. The doctor walked away without answering us. This was it! We had had enough of this nonsense! Why was he behaving so malevolently toward us like this?

Chapter 9

We talked on the way home from his office about the doctor's behavior. DeWayne was furious! He said as soon as we got home he was going to write him a long letter stating our concerns, questioning the information we had been given about my medication and dosages, and stating that if he could not answer us truthfully, we would find someone else. He also told him that we would not cancel our son's appointment and we would be rescheduling my next treatment for after his hospital stay. He then took the letter that same day and left it at the doctor's office.

Later that evening I was very ill again. As before, DeWayne made me a bed on the bathroom floor and lay down with me. Like the first treatment, it continued for a few hours. I was distraught about this new bout of upchucking everything. Nevertheless, this time, DeWayne and I stood together to get me through it. The nausea did not last as long as before. However, it was two days before I was able to keep anything down. I continued to lose weight and get weaker. All the same, we considered it a victory that we made it through without having to go into the hospital. I still had to go in the next few days and have daily shots to keep my white count up, however.

The next week we met with the doctor about the letter and had a long conversation. He wrote down on a sheet of paper what I was taking and how much. The numbers did not agree with what he had told us in the treatment room the week before. I pointed to it and told him that this was the first time he ever detailed for us what I was taking. He said he had expected us to read all the material that he had given us at the beginning. My husband reminded him that while the papers listed the three original chemo drugs he wanted to give me, they did not list dosages, or any of the changes he had made since the treatments began.

They also did not address the real problem. The treatment was making me so sick and weak that it was putting my life and health in danger. At this point, instead of depression, I was fuming.

Finally, the doctor suggested a different treatment. Instead of the remaining three IV treatments normally administered in three to four hours, he wanted me to spend twenty-four hours in the hospital where they would give me a slow drip of chemo. He hoped that by slowing the treatment, it would eliminate the nausea. Just two more of those treatments, and I would be done. Nonetheless, by this time, both of us were extremely frustrated. I, myself, was so upset that I wanted to just stop and give up this whole chaos. I felt I could not go through another treatment. The horror of another hospital stay was unbearable. I just could not do it.

DeWayne and I talked on the way home from the doctor's office. Sobbing, I told him my feelings. He pulled into the church parking lot, which is not that far from our house. He stopped the car and pulled me next to him. He spoke very gently and encouragingly. He said he did not know the answer to what we should do, but one thing was for sure, he was not going to lose me. In between his tears, he told me how much he loved me more than anything and was not going to let the devil have me. God was going to give us an answer. He then decided that when we got home we would call our Care-Net couple again for help.

Once we arrived home, we called our Care-Net couple and talked with them. They suggested talking to our family physician about what was going on. They prayed with us for guidance and wisdom.

We talked to our family doctor, who is a spirit-filled Christian. Our family doctor is one who deeply cares about his patients. He has a special gift with people. He always takes time with each patient and listens to what they have to say about what is bothering them. He would joke with his patients to help them feel better and to help them keep calm. We would always leave his office feeling better than when we did when we got there. He listened very intently and was extremely upset on how we were treated by both oncologists. We talked for an hour. We found out that he had never received any reports from this oncologist, which upset us. I told him that I would tell the oncologist receptionist that I wanted reports sent to him on a regular basis. Our doctor suggested going ahead with the two treatments. If I am sick, it would only be two more times and then it would be over. We asked him about referring us to another doctor for the final treatments, but when he checked, he learned that because we had already changed doctor's once, my insurance would not cover another change in doctors. Our physician prayed with us for wisdom with the oncologist before we left.

Chapter 10

One more time we talked to the oncologist, and again he suggested another different treatment. I also kept in contact with the receptionist to make sure my family doctor was getting reports. I thought maybe now, after the letter and conversation, the doctor would start being truthful with us.

I would start having radiation treatments along with six small weekly chemo treatments. It was supposed to be the best chemo for breast cancer. Now why he did not suggest this in the first place, we do not know. Therefore, I proceeded with this new treatment. The doctor had also started me on a new medication to reduce my hot flashes without changing any medication that I was already taking. God spoke to me to read the insert that came with the medicine. I realized that I was about to take the same type of medication that was similar to what I was already taking. Not only was the medication supposed to help stop hot flashes, but it was also an anti-depressant. I called the nurse at the office, asked her about it, and she said yes, do not take the old anti-depressant any more. God had stepped in again and saved me from overdosing myself.

I had to go into Flint by the hospital to get these treatments, because the doctor's second office that I had been going to did not have the equipment for radiation. This office had three oncologists and one radiologist. I did not get ill from the chemo, but I was very fatigued for the next three days. Now I had to take one day at a time and believe for that day when I would be through with the treatments. I had to go twice a week after the chemo treatment in order to get two shots to raise my white count. Radiation was every day for six weeks. The lady tech in radiation was a Christian. We got along very well. We talked about the Lord and home schooling. She was home schooling her daughter like I was home schooling my son. The radiologist doctor was a woman and very informative. She was very sweet and kind. She had no trouble in answering all our questions. She described in detail how the radiation worked and took us on a tour of the treatment room. I would have the whole breast radiated and then, the last four days of the therapy, I would have just the place where the tumor was removed radiated. When we left there, we knew what I would be facing. This brought great peace of mind. Later, when I was burned from the treatments, she gave me special medicine to help heal the burn quickly and started me on the other radiation so I would not keep burning in the same place. During this time, my hair started growing back. It seemed slow at first, but then I noticed that every week it was a new length. It was getting longer and longer.

Still, at the same time, DeWayne and I stood believing God's Word. I had to make the decision whether to believe God would do what He said in the Bible or not. I had chosen to believe God. Why would He say the things in the Bible about long life and healing if they were not true? I put myself in God's hands and said, "I receive the Word of God for me."

I started counting down the weeks of the chemo treatments, telling myself four more to go, three, two, one. I also kept myself busy with what I could do, which was home schooling my son and working on cross-stitch (needlepoint). I did not need to stand or walk around to do these things. Everyone in my household helped me by doing things that I could not do, like washing the dishes, cleaning the house, and sweeping the floors. Trying to do even these simple activities drained me. I was more or less confined to my recliner. My sons made me breakfast and lunch and then would bring them to me. My husband cooked dinner and brought that to me. I did not have to move much. I did not like not being able to do any activity, and as soon as the treatments were over, I planned to start working out to help get my body back in shape.

The time came for my last treatment. I met with a different specialist since the one I had been seeing was not there. I told him my six treatments were up. He said I was supposed to have twelve treatments. Again, we found out the other doctor had lied to us. We talked to our Care-Net couple again. Now I had to decide whether to continue with the treatments or end it. I was through with the doctor who would not tell us the truth. Nevertheless, at the same time, I did not want to give any place to the devil by not completing the treatments. Our couple prayed with us for guidance. I decided to go ahead and finish with the last six treatments. I would just have to start over and count down once again, but this time I knew I would finally be done. DeWayne supported my decision. He also supported me every week by taking me to my chemo treatments and to one of the days to get my shot. My daughters took two of the days to take me to my radiation treatments. My oldest son went with me to my second shot day so I could have an arm to give me support. My walking was a little unstable.

Chapter 11

DeWayne came with me as he always did when I had to go get my shot for my white count. An older gentleman sat next to me and started a conversation with us. He asked if we knew the Lord and we said yes. We asked him how he came to know the Lord, and he told us that he was on an airplane carrier in the Pacific Ocean during World War II. He said explosions were going on all around him. He suddenly realized that if he died, he would go to hell. He wanted to make sure he was right with the Lord, got saved right there on the carrier, and had been serving the Lord ever since then. He told us about the doctor he was seeing and that the doctor believed in God. DeWayne and I had met him once all ready. He was the one that told us I was originally supposed to get twelve treatments. We had liked him because he had a wonderful and caring attitude. The doctor was a little upset that we had been told wrong information about the number of treatments I was supposed to have. We decided that he was the one we were going to see from now on. The older gent also told us that most of the nurses there were Christians.

I had a favorite nurse that would give me my treatments because she was always friendly, loved people and cared for them. She was also very good at her job. She never had any trouble inserting the needle into my passport. Sometimes when she was not there and another nurse would try to start my treatment, that nurse would have trouble with getting the needle into my passport. Once during one of my chemo treatments, I watched my favorite nurse as she took a patient and explained all the drugs he would be getting during his chemotherapy and all the information, the medicines that he was to take and what they were for. Everything that he needed to know about his treatments —she took him through it all. She was very thorough. I was impressed and wished someone had done that for me. I also watched this one doctor, the one I liked. He came back to the chemo room often, talked with the patients, and answered their questions. He was very interested in helping the people. I never saw my original physician in the chemo room.

At last, I finished all the treatments and met with the new doctor. He was very good and explained the follow up check-ups. I would come back for an examination every three months, then every six months and then once a year. I would not need to take a chemotherapy pill every day. I do not know the name of it. He did tell us, but it was one of those big, long Latin names. Since I did not need it, I did not bother to try to remember it. We were impressed with the information this specialist was giving us. He was thorough and complete. Finally, DeWayne and I felt at peace with this new oncologist.

Chapter 12

Where there is no vision, the people perish;...

Proverbs 29:18 (KJV)

At church, Pastor had been talking about vision and goals. I realized that I needed that too. I needed goals for my life. Therefore, I started planning. The video department was going through a transition. We were going to be getting new equipment, because the equipment we had was all very old and out-dated. Moreover, it was wearing out. I kept the cameras and video recorders running by constantly repairing them. Most of the repair work I could do myself. If it got a little more complicated than I could deal with, I took it to a repair service that helped me tremendously and got it done quickly. They had the equipment repaired in time for the next service. All we could do for the time being with the videotapes was to sell them through our bookstore that we had at the church. We wanted to get our services on television so we could reach more people. I had a lot of research to do. I needed to find studio cameras, a mixer board, monitors, a digital recorder, and units that would tell which individual camera was recording. Besides that, there was a lot I wanted to do with my life. I wanted to produce and direct TV shows, write novels, write and direct plays, and write musicals. One thing that I really wanted to do was to write and direct a movie. I had also wanted to produce and direct a musical at our church. That was a dream and I was not about to give up. God had given me the name of the musical that I was supposed to do one night at midnight. I was so excited that I started doing research on it. It was "Godspell." I shared it with DeWayne, and he helped me with ideas, and so forth. There was a lot of work to do to prepare for it. Since I had never done anything quite like this before, it took several months.

Chapter 13

I started gaining weight, pound by pound, and getting stronger and stronger. DeWayne and I worked out on my son's Bowflex, a home gym. Every few weeks we had to up the weight because it was getting too easy for me. Every week I was getting better and better. My hair was now at a length, about two inches, which I was comfortable with for going out in public, so I stopped wearing the wig. Not only was my hair a beautiful length, but also it was very soft, thick, and wavy. It had never been that way before. My weight settled at about one hundred thirty-five pounds. The added weight well-fitted my tall frame and made me look terrific. In addition, I had had eczema on my hands as long as I can remember. I was always very self-conscious about them because they looked so ugly. Suddenly it was all gone. For the first time in my life, I was free of eczema. My hands looked wonderful. God had taken the bad, turned it around, and had given me more than I had ever had previously.

I also had more energy than I had had in months. Finally, I was able to do what I had wanted to do for awhile. That was to clean my house and rid it of junk, things that I had not used in years, clothes that were worn out and did not fit any more. Books and old papers that were not needed were thrown away. It felt good to be busy after months of not being able to do anything. I even helped my daughters organize their house, but at the same time, I kept finding things in my own home to clean out. Moreover, I was back working in the Video Department. I was happy.

Then came the day when I had to have tests, mammogram and pap smears, to make sure no cancer could be found in my body. DeWayne and I agreed together and our Care-Net couple prayed with us. We saw the new doctor and got the results saying no more cancer. The nurses were running their hands through my hair, amazed at how soft my hair was. My favorite nurse asked me if my hair had always been like this, and I told her no. A week later, the radiologist sent a report to me with the same results. No evidence of cancer found. I told Pastor, and he announced it to the congregation the next Sunday morning after I got the results. The people of our church went nuts. Everyone was jumping up and down and screaming for joy. For at least five minutes, the place went wild. I had not realized until that moment how many people had been furiously praying for me. All I could do was stand there with tears streaming down my face, praising God. It was wonderful to have so many people rejoicing with us.

The next week the oncologist had my passport taken out, saying I would not need it again. I went into the hospital with the prayers of agreement of DeWayne and our Care-Net couple that everything would go smoothly, quickly, and with no complications. That is what happened. I had a different surgeon that took out the port this time. He was friendly, talkative, and encouraging. He kept telling me that if I felt any sharp pain to tell him and he would give me some more numbing medicine. However, I did not need it. He and the nurses kept talking to me with small talk and fun. Everyone was laughing and having a good time while I just lay there with him digging in my arm trying to find the tube. However, he got the port out quickly and sewed me up. I even got the chance to see what it looked like. He explained how it worked. It was very interesting. It was a small gray box, about one inch high and two inches long, with two small buttons on the top with a long white tube coming out of the bottom. It seemed too big to fit in my arm without me noticing the size, but I had no idea. The buttons were where the nurses put in the IV's. The long white tube went into the major vein.

The whole episode was finally over. The surgery, the chemotherapy, the radiation treatments were finally finished. It had been very traumatic and frightening. Nevertheless, I got through it with a lot of prayer and a lot of support from my husband, my Pastor, the people of my church, and my Care-Net couple. With their support and God's Word, I made it through.

Chapter 14

People will tell others *to believe God, stand on His Word, and say the Word.* They make it sound so easy, but it is not. It is a battle, a battle with the mind — silencing the negative thoughts, putting only God's Word in its place, making goals and visions for one's life. I did not want to sound negative, but not too many people would tell the things that happened to them or the things they went through. I want people to know the trials we went through and the victories we won going through the trials. Our Pastor was always saying pass through the trial, do not stand in the middle of it. When we were in the doctor's office, we were always surrounded by death and negative words. We had to pray to keep ourselves covered with God's Word against these oppressions. Every time people hear the phrase breast cancer, they think death. We could not allow ourselves to think that. Was it easy to just stop the negative words, thoughts, and surroundings? No, it took determination. It was not easy, but it was necessary.

Every time I went to church during my treatments, it seemed like our music team always led us in victory songs. Those songs helped build my faith and spirit. Again, God led the people of my church to agree with me even though they did not know they were doing it. Pastor's teaching was constantly building me with more of God's Word of victory and authority. He probably was not aware of how much he was helping me, but I soaked up every word, every teaching.

As Pastor taught me, I had to see God's Word inside me. I had to agree with the Word. I needed to say what the Word of God had to say, and God would back it up. He would not back up what I say, but He would back up what He says. Satan will back up the negative words. He does not have any trouble doing that. For God to deny His Word, He would have to deny His name. God takes great stock in His Word. I could base my life on the Word of God. Therefore, I needed to keep saying the Word of God. I needed to keep the Word of God on my lips.

The Lord had made a covenant. His Word would not change. What He said is true. I had to believe what He said. I could not decide one day that God's Word is true and I was going to follow it, and then the next day decide that it was not for me. If God said He would do it, then He will do it. I had to choose whether I was going to believe Him or not.

I spoke the Word of God, the scriptures mentioned above, plus a few others. Reading the Bible aloud and saying the scriptures aloud every time fear or doubt would try to enter my mind helped keep me under control. I make it sound easy, but it was not. I also knew that I was not going to allow satan to win. God said that I was healed by His stripes. That is my right. God said that He would perform His Word. My husband and I spoke the Word of God together. We never spoke anything negative. We spoke only the Word of God concerning my health. After all the tests and surgery, there is not a trace of cancer.

The question I asked myself was, "Why not just believe that God would heal me?" That is what I did. God did heal me with His Word. The surgery and tests confirmed that God's Word works. God uses doctors, too.

I am a survivor of cancer because of God's Word and the prayers of people who believed in not giving up and standing with us and with me. Our Care-Net couple was not going to let me fail. Their help and tenacity along with the Word kept me going. I passed through the trial. I did not stay in the middle.

Chapter 15

The next three chapters are notes I took while listening to Pastor Barancik. They reached deep in my heart to help me in every situation and circumstance that I've been through. These are truths that will help you out of events that satan likes to bring up against you. Open your heart and mind while you are reading, and will set you free.

So what is all this standing on the Word of God and speaking the Word of God? It's called faith. It's all about faith. Faith is so important. In the middle of our struggle, we have something to obtain our healing. There's never any shortage of faith available to us, and it's faith that we need to get from the sickness to the healing. But to get there, we need to change our thinking. We need to get our thinking off the circumstances and get it on faith. Faith will change anything.

"The heavens are the Lord's heavens, but the earth has He given to the children of men." Psalms 155:16 (AMP) The Lord gave us the authority over the earth. Sometimes we are looking to God to change the situations, and God said we need to take authority over it according to Genesis chapter 1. He told us to take dominion over it. That is why

faith is so important, because faith will overtake any circumstance or situation and cause us to be blessed. Faith is our avenue to get what we see as our hopes or dreams to manifest in our life. God's Word can do it. Faith can make the difference.

"For whatever is born of God is victorious over the world; and this is the victory that conquers the world, even our faith. Who is it that is victorious over (that conquers) the world but he who believes that Jesus is the Son of God — who adheres to, trusts in and relies [on that fact]? 1 John 5:4-5 (AMP) If we have faith for it, it will overcome anything we face. There's not one problem or situation that can't be fixed if we have faith. How do we get that overcoming faith? If we are born of God, we have that overcoming faith. There's nothing that faith can't answer. *"If you live in Me — abide vitally united to Me — and My words remain in you and continue to live in your hears, ask whatever you will and it shall be done for you."* John 15:7 (AMP) Faith overcomes the world. If we can get into a place of faith, we already have the answer.

"Truly, I tell you, whoever says to this mountain, Be lifted up and thrown into the sea! And does not doubt at all in his heart, but believes that what he says will take place, it will be done for him." Mark 11:23 (AMP) This means faith will work for everyone. No one is denied access to faith. God didn't say the circumstances would obey Him. He said they would obey us. Sometimes we say, "God, remove the mountain; I believe You can do it." He says, "Ok, you (meaning us) can do it." This scripture verse didn't say the mountain would obey Him; it said it would obey you (us). That's faith. Reality begins in the world of faith, not after we see it. Reality is what happens in the world of faith. We see it in the world of faith, the supernatural. Some might say, "I'll believe it when I see it." That's doubt. Faith is, "I believe I receive it now."

"Therefore [because He stooped so low], God has highly exalted Him and has freely bestowed on Him the name that is above every name, That in (at) the name of Jesus every knee should (must) bow, in heaven and on earth and under the earth, And every tongue [frankly and openly] confess and acknowledge that Jesus Christ is Lord, to the glory of God the Father." Philippians 2:9-11. (AMP) Everything has a name — cancer, lack, sickness, etc. We must make that name bow to the name of Jesus.

Chapter 16

"For we walk by faith [that is, we regulate our lives and conduct ourselves by our conviction or belief respecting man's relationship to God and divine things, with trust and holy fervor; thus we walk] not by sight or appearance."

2 Corinthians 5:7 (AMP)

"Because if you acknowledge and confess with your lips that Jesus is Lord and in your heart believe (adhere to, trust in and rely on the truth) that God raised Him from the dead, you will be saved." Romans 10:9 (AMP)

There are two principles in this verse, believing and confessing. Believing and confessing is another way to exercise faith. What are you believing? What are you saying? *"For with the heart a person believes (adheres to, trusts in and relies on Christ) and so is justified (declared righteous, acceptable to God), and with the mouth he confesses — declares openly and speaks out freely his faith — and confirms [his] salvation."* Romans 10:10 (AMP) "I believe that I have my healing because by His stripes I was healed." Then I confess it. "Body, you are healed in Jesus' name." With the heart, the man believes, and with the mouth he confesses. We have to say something. As Christians, we must understand this principle of confession. You may say, "Well, I'm not going to say something if I don't see it." If you only say what you see, then what you see is all you'll ever get. What do you believe? Can you say it? In the Kingdom of God, it's different. You must say it first, then you see it second. You believe it, you see it in the spirit, you say it, and then you see it manifest. That's how God operates.

"*So then faith cometh by hearing, and hearing by the word of God.*" Romans 10:17 (KJV) When we allow ourselves to hear the Word of God by reading it, by quoting it, by memorizing it, through meditating on it, through listening to it preached, listening to it on CD, you really hear the Word. Faith comes from the Word of God. Faith comes to you by truly hearing the Word of God. If you see it in the Bible, you can have faith to expect it in your life. Jesus healed people in the Bible, so you can have faith to be healed today.

"*Death and life are in the power of the tongue: and they that love it shall eat the fruit thereof.*" Proverbs 18:21 (KJV) What are we speaking? If we speak the negative, we are going to eat the negative. If we speak the positive, we are going to eat the positive. Go back to Mark 11:23. What does it say? It says, "*say unto this mountain, Be thou removed, and be thou cast into the sea; and shall not doubt in his heart, but shall believe that those things which he saith shall come to pass; he shall have whatsoever he saith.*" (KJV) Speak to the situation; don't doubt in your heart; believe what you say, and you shall have it. You have to say it. Faith comes by hearing the Word of God. That's why we can say faith comes to us by hearing ourselves saying the Word of God.

"I will give you the keys of the kingdom of heaven, and whatever you bind — that is, declare to be improper and unlawful — on earth must be already bound in heaven; and whatever you loose on earth — declare lawful — must be what is already loosed in heaven." Matthew 16:19 (AMP) What is bound in heaven? Sickness, lack, cancer, etc. are not allowed in heaven. Then we know that we can make it so here, too. What's loosed in heaven? Peace, joy, health, prosperity, etc. is what is loosed in heaven, so we can loose health in our lives. Bring what's loosed in heaven to you. If it's lawful in heaven, then we can have it here.

Chapter 17

"My son, attend to my words; consent and submit to my sayings. Let them not depart from your sight; keep them in the center of your heart. For they are life to those who find them, healing and health to all their flesh."

Proverbs 4:20-22 (AMP)

What is planted in your heart? Just going to a church that believes that you can be cancer free will not heal you of cancer. It's what you have planted in your heart that makes the difference. Have you planted fear, unbelief, doubt, or wrong speaking? Or have you planted what the Word of God says? Are you saying, "This faith stuff doesn't work?" Then, of course, it is not going to work for you. This Word stuff works, but it has to be in the right place, in your ear, in your eyes, and in your heart. The promise is that if we have it in our ear, in what our eyes are focused on, and in what is in our heart, the Word is life to all our flesh. Find a promise in the Word of God that applies to you, and speak it to get the result you want. The more you speak it, the more it will get into your heart.

Before the Word can be life and health, it must be heard, received and attended to. We have to hear it; we have to receive it; and we have to attend to it. Hear the Word of God by speaking it. Then don't let the Word depart from your eyes. Are you looking at the symptoms of the sickness, or are you looking at what the Word says about your healing? You may say, "I know the Word is true." That's not going to do it. That's not faith. That's just affirming that the Word is true. That's a false faith. "Yes, I know what the Word says." But then if you turn around and say, "Did you see how bad it is? Do you see what is happening?" That is not faith. You do not have the Word planted powerfully in your heart. It is so easy to look at the symptoms, but if you want victory, then you must not let your eyes depart from the Word. It's not easy, but if you want victory, you must do it.

How do you attend to the Word? Look at the answer. What does the Word say? "But I'm going through sickness." What does the Word say? Are you looking at the problem, or are you looking at the answer? You may be trying to believe God for the answer, but God says, "Look at the answer."

"The sower sows the Word. The ones along the path are those who have the Word sown [in their hearts], but when they hear, Satan comes at once and (by force) takes away the message which is sown in them. And in the same way the ones sown upon stony ground are those who, when they hear the Word, at once receive and accept and welcome it with joy; and they have no real root in themselves, and so they endure for a little while, then when trouble or persecution arises on account of the Word, they immediately are offended — become displeased, indignant, resentful; and they stumble and fall away. And the ones sown among the thorns are others who hear the Word, Then the cares and anxieties of the world, and distractions of

the age, and the pleasure and delight and false glamour and deceitfulness of riches, and the craving and passionate desire for other things creep in and choke and suffocate the Word, and it becomes fruitless. And those that were sown on the good (well-adapted) soil are the ones who hear the Word, and receive and accept and welcome it and bear fruit, some thirty times as much as was sown, some sixty times as much, and some [even] a hundred times as much." Mark 4:14-20 (AMP)

Keep the Word in the center of your heart. Your heart is like the ground. You plant seed in it. You've got to let it grow. The Word is like seed. You must let it grow in your heart. What have you planted in your heart? Are you saying, "It's not working?" If so, what did you plant in your heart? You may say, "Oh, I love the Lord," but the Word is not sown in your heart. You may say, "Oh, I'm believing Him." Ok, what did you do in the last twenty-four hours? What has your thinking been about? What has your talking been about? What have you been looking at? What have you been hearing? And what have you been repeating? Whatever you have been doing is in your heart. You may say, "Oh, just because I talk about it doesn't mean it's in my heart." Oh, yes, it does. Jesus said, *"For out of the abundance of the heart his mouth speaks."* Luke 6:45b (NKJV) You must attend to the Word. Hear it, hear it. When all that doubt and unbelief comes, stop yourself and say the Word. Keep saying it.

The enemy does not play favorites. He will mess things up in your life. Have you been saying, "This isn't working. I've tried it?" No, you don't TRY the Word, you DO the Word. It's the enemy that will try you. You will either try the Word or you won't. Don't feed on doubt. If you can get the Word centered in your heart, don't worry about it. It's going to produce. It will produce. We don't have to make the Word work. The process is in the seed of the Word. The Word will work. *"The Word of God, which is effectually at work in you who believe — exercising its [superhuman] power in those who adhere to and trust in and rely on it."* 1 Thessalonians 2:13b (AMP) *"To this end I also labor, striving according to His working which works in me mightily."* Colossians 1:29 (NKJV) *"Now to Him who is able to do exceedingly abundantly above all that we ask or think, according to the power that works in us,"* Ephesians 3:20 (NKJV)

You may still be saying, "This isn't working." No, what you are saying is you're not working it in you. You haven't been planting. Hear the Word, put your focus on the Word, put the Word in your heart. The Word will work. How do you get the Word in your heart? Read it, meditate on it, memorize it, quote it, or sing it. The Word does work. We don't have to make it work, it just works. But what are you sowing in your heart? What are you planting in your heart?

Chapter 18

For us to believe that God's Word will work for us, we must first be sure that we have a relationship with Him. I am talking about a relationship, not religion. If you are just attending church because someone else is, that is not going to get you to heaven or make the Word of God work for you. Our relationship with God comes after we confess with our mouth that Jesus is Lord and believe in our heart that God raised Him from the dead (Romans 10:9). Let us take a moment and read some scriptures to make sure of our relationship (covenant) with God.

> *For the wages of sin is death; but the gift of God is eternal life through Jesus Christ our Lord.*
>
> Romans 6:23 (KJV)

Eternal life is a free gift, but everyone who has sinned has earned spiritual death. God wants to give us eternal life, but we are not good enough to get it. If we think that we are going to heaven if we live a life without stealing or hurting people, it will not work. If we think we are going to heaven by being good or just going to church every week or every now and then, it will not work.

> *Therefore if any man be in Christ, he is a new creature;*
> *old things are passed away; behold, all things are become*
> *new.*   2 Corinthians 5:17 (KJV)

We become a new being, a new creature, once we have accepted Christ. Everything that was in the past is past. We are brand new. The old person we were is no more. Nevertheless, you say, "What is wrong with the way I am? I like my life just as it is." Fine, but that will not get you into heaven. You say, "I can think about heaven later. I've got time." Really? Without God, you may be wiped out tomorrow. You have no control over your life until you become a Christian and learn how to walk in the superior life. Once you become a Christian, you have this brand new life, a better life, the superior life. You like the way you are living now, but what if you could have a superior life? You can, by receiving Jesus as Lord and Savior. You may think that you have no sin, but everyone does. How do we get rid of sin? How do we get started in this superior life?

> *For he hath made him to be sin for us, who knew no sin;*
> *that we might be made the righteousness of God in him.*
>   2 Corinthians 5:21 (KJV)

Jesus traded our sin for His righteousness. There is only one way we can encounter His righteousness and have eternal life. That is by receiving Jesus as Savior and Lord by Faith. This is how to reach out for the superior life.

> *That if thou shalt confess with thy mouth the Lord Jesus, and shalt believe in thine heart that God hath raised him from the dead, thou shalt be saved. For with the heart man believeth unto righteousness; and with the mouth confession is made unto salvation.*
>
> Romans 10:9-10 (KJV)

Faith just believes what God said is true. Receiving Jesus as Savior means understanding that Jesus exchanged places with us to make amends for our sin and give us His righteousness. We know that without Jesus we would never go to Heaven. Receiving Jesus as Lord means feeling sorry about our sins, turning around, and beginning to do what Jesus wants us to do, making Him the authority over our lives.

Pray this prayer: "Lord Jesus, forgive me for my sins and come into my life. Be my Lord and Savior. Take control of my life. I place You first in my life. I ask this in the name of Jesus. Amen."

Now be sure to find other Christians who will help you grow and will show you how to live in this supreme life. You will need a church that teaches the Word of God and shows you how to operate it in your life.

If you need prayer for deliverance from cancer, pray this prayer: "I take authority over cancer right now in Jesus' name. Cancer, you are a name. At the name of Jesus, every knee shall bow, and you must bow to the name of Jesus. I bind you, curse you from the root, and tell you to be gone. Dissolve in the name of Jesus. You have no more power over me. Mind and body, you will adhere to the Word of God. In the name of Jesus, body, you are healed, because Jesus said that by His stripes I am healed. Thank you, Lord. Amen."

Remember to read and say God's Word daily to keep control over your thoughts. If you have not received Jesus as Lord and Savior, then this prayer will not work for you. To have the authority of God's Word, you must be in God's kingdom by becoming a Christian. Every Christian has had to accept Jesus as Lord and Savior. There is no way of getting around it. Do the smart thing. Receive Jesus. You will never regret it.

ABOUT THE AUTHOR

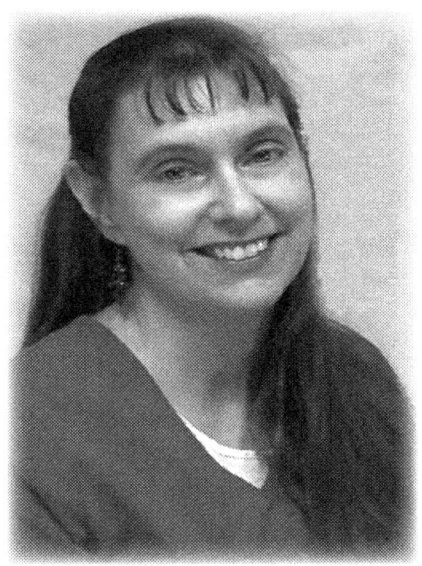

Patty was the director of the TV/Video Department at Faith City Church (formally Faith Fellowship Ministries) in Fenton, Michigan. With the Video Department now in transition while waiting for new equipment, she helps with recording the services on audio CD's.

Patty is also producer and director of the church's new theater group, "Royal Court Productions." The vision for Royal Court is to take back the media and theater for Christ and to reach our community for Jesus. This is a theater group geared for family and Christian entertainment by performing musicals, dramas, comedies, and some original productions. Her husband, DeWayne, supports and works beside her in the theater. Both are accomplished playwrights and directors. Their first production, "Godspell" was performed in 2003 with great results. Both are also involved in the local community theater, Fenton Village Players.

DeWayne and Patty are proud parents of 4 children: 2 girls and 2 boys plus 1 grandson and a baby girl on the way Both daughters are married with one of them living across from DeWayne and Patty. One son is attending an online college course through Westwood Campus. The last son graduated Valedictorian in 2005 from Good Heritage Academy.

If you would like to write Patty, address your letters to:

DeWayne and Patty Coons
c/o Faith City Church
2084 W Thompson Rd
Fenton, MI 48430

She would love to hear from you, especially if you have received Jesus as Lord and Savior.